Iyengar Yoga with Rope Wall for Beginners

By Smith J. Offor

I0454409

Table of Contents

Introduction

Iyengar Yoga stands as a gateway to holistic well-being, especially for beginners aspiring to shed those extra pounds. It transcends the physical realm of mere weight loss, diving deep into the realms of mental peace, emotional stability, and physical harmony.

Unraveling the Essence of Iyengar Yoga

The core philosophy of Iyengar Yoga is precision and alignment in postures (asanas). Rooted in Hatha Yoga, this style emphasizes controlled movement and attention to detail, making it ideal for novices aiming for weight management.

Key Elements of Iyengar Yoga Practice

Accessibility: Unlike intense forms, Iyengar Yoga is accessible to all, irrespective of age or fitness level.

Guidance: Iyengar Yoga Beginners benefit from instructor-led sessions to grasp foundational techniques.

Attention to Detail: Focus on posture alignment ensures safety and efficacy in practice.

Use of Props: Props like blocks, belts, and blankets aid beginners in mastering asanas with ease and reduce the risk of injury.

How Iyengar Yoga Supports Weight Loss
Precision and Calorie Burn

Iyengar Yoga's deliberate and structured approach engages muscle groups deeply, enhancing calorie expenditure and facilitating weight loss.

Precision in Asanas
Each posture is meticulously crafted, ensuring optimal engagement of muscles, amplifying the calorie-burning process.

Mind-Body Harmony
The practice of Iyengar Yoga instills mindfulness, awareness, and emotional balance, curtailing

overeating tendencies born out of stress or emotional triggers.

Stress Reduction

The integration of meditative postures aids in stress reduction, minimizing unhealthy eating patterns linked to emotional turmoil.

Metabolism and Hormonal Balance

The precision-based practice, coupled with breath control, promotes better metabolic function and hormonal equilibrium, contributing to effective weight management.

Beginners' Guide to Embracing Iyengar Yoga

Essential Tips for Novice Practitioners

Consistency Matters: Practice regularly to observe progress and reap the benefits effectively.

Guidance is Key: Seek guidance from a skilled instructor to ensure correct posture and technique.

Equip Yourself: Basic yoga gear like a yoga mat and comfortable attire suffice for a home practice.

Breathe Right: Emphasize the significance of deep and controlled breathing throughout your practice.

Listen to Your Body: Progress at your pace, respecting your body's limitations to prevent injuries.

Challenge and Grow: Gradually introduce challenges to your routine to ensure consistent progress.

Prep and Cool Down: Initiate sessions with a warm-up and conclude with calming poses to ease transitions.

Frequently Asked Questions

Is Iyengar Yoga suitable for weight loss beginners?

Absolutely! Iyengar Yoga's precise approach and accessible techniques cater perfectly to beginners, ensuring a safe yet effective weight loss journey.

Can I practice Iyengar Yoga at home without an instructor?

While it's feasible, starting under the supervision ofan experienced instructor is recommended for correct posture and alignment.

How does Iyengar Yoga differ from other yoga styles in aiding weight loss?

Iyengar Yoga's focus on alignment, use of props, and emphasis on detail sets it apart, ensuring a safe and structured weight loss practice.

How soon can one expect to see weight loss results with Iyengar Yoga?

Consistency and dedication are key. With regular practice and a balanced diet, visible results can be witnessed in a few weeks.

Are there specific Iyengar Yoga poses that target weight loss?

While the practice doesn't emphasize specific poses for weight loss, its precise alignment in various postures effectively engages muscle groups, contributing to calorie burn and weight management.

Does Iyengar Yoga aid only in weight loss, or are there other benefits?

Apart from weight loss, Iyengar Yoga fosters mental peace, physical strength, and emotional balance, making it a holistic approach to well-being.

How long should a beginner practice Iyengar Yoga for optimal weight loss?

Starting with shorter sessions of 20-30 minutes, gradually increasing duration as one progresses, can yield effective weight loss results.

Can I combine other exercises with Iyengar Yoga for better weight loss outcomes?

Certainly! Combining yoga with other exercises like cardio or strength training can further enhance weight loss outcomes.

Can Iyengar Yoga help in emotional eating and stress-related weight gain?

Absolutely! The mindfulness and stress-relieving benefits of Iyengar Yoga can aid in curbing emotional eating habits and managing stress-induced weight gain.

Is there a recommended dietary pattern to complement Iyengar Yoga for weight loss?

While Iyengar Yoga promotes mindful eating, coupling it with a balanced diet rich in fruits, vegetables, and whole grains amplifies weight loss benefits.

Incorporating Iyengar Yoga into your daily routine serves as an effective pathway to weight management and holistic wellness. With its precision, accessibility, and holistic approach, this yoga style promises a fulfilling journey towards a healthier you.

The Versatility and Health Benefits of Yoga Wall Ropes

Understanding the Origins of Yoga Wall Ropes

Yoga Wall Ropes, initially introduced by BKS Iyengar, hold a fascinating history rooted in enhancing the yoga practice. Inspired by nature's design, these ropes draw parallels to the unique joint preservation mechanism observed in bats and sloths that evade arthritis through consistent inverted postures.

Unlocking the Health Benefits

Harnessing Gravity for Holistic Wellness

The utilization of gravity as a resistance tool via the ropes amplifies the depth and extension of traditional yoga postures. Mimicking the upside-down suspension of bats and sloths, this technique alleviates joint stress, fostering profound muscular-skeletal stretching.

Promoting Spine Health and Relief

Yoga rope poses are instrumental in spine health by offering traction, relieving vertebral disc pressure, easing compressed nerves, and inducing a tranquil state of mind. Additionally, they facilitate a deep organic body opening, enhancing extracellular fluid flow to nourish organs and tissues.

Exploring Variants of Yoga Rope Wall Systems
A Diverse Spectrum of Rope Wall Setups

Ranging from basic eye screw installations to elaborate ball and socket joints, these setups vary in complexity and functionality, catering to diverse preferences and spaces.

Eye Screw Setup: Cost-Effective and Simple

Construction: Involves 2" eye screws fitted into wall studs with precision, necessitating expert installation for optimal results.

Connectivity: Utilizes climbing grade karabina clips to affix ropes, enhancing ease of attachment and detachment.

Design and Measurement Considerations

Customization: The setup allows tailor-made adjustments, including personalized rope heights suiting individual practitioners.

Spatial Requirements: Ensures adequate clearance for horizontal poses, optimizing user comfort and safety.

Premade Rope Wall Solutions

Innovative Mechanisms: The Great Yoga Wall offers premade systems employing ball and socket joints for seamless attachment of ropes.

Custom Installations: Services like Socal Yoga Walls offer nationwide custom installations, offering accessibility and convenience.

Procuring Yoga Wall Ropes: A Comprehensive Guide

Accessing Readily Available Solutions

Online Platforms: Platforms such as Yoga Props or Tools for Yoga provide premade rope options suitable for diverse requirements.

Local Suppliers: Personalized ropes tailored to specifications can be acquired from trusted local suppliers, ensuring quality and customization.

Crafting Your Own Ropes: A DIY Approach

Material Insights: Recommendations and insights for choosing the right rope material and thickness, optimizing grip and comfort.

Procurement Tips: Suggestions for acquiring suitable ropes, including ideal suppliers and potential drawbacks of certain materials.

Safely Embracing Rope Wall Practices

The Imperative of Professional Guidance

Qualified Instructors: Advocating for trained and experienced instructors to navigate the complexities and safety nuances of rope wall practices.

Expertise Criteria: Suggested qualifications include years of personal practice and robust understanding to avert potential risks.

Resources and Expert Guidance

Comprehensive Learning Tools

Educational Materials: Books like "Yoga a Gem for Women" by Geeta Iyengar and instructional PDFs offer in-depth insights and guidance.

Video Tutorials: Online resources like YouTube videos featuring prominent teachers illustrate practical rope wall practices effectively.

Frequently Asked Questions

How do Yoga Wall Ropes aid joint health?

Yoga ropes leverage gravity for joint relief, offering traction to alleviate vertebral pressure and nurture overall spine health.

Are premade rope wall systems customizable?

Yes, solutions like The Great Yoga Wall offer customizable setups, ensuring adaptability to varied spaces and individual needs.

What precautions should one consider before practicing on the yoga wall?

Prioritize seeking professional guidance to prevent hazards like falls, overstretching, and potential muscle strains, ensuring a safe practice environment.

Can beginners explore yogarope practices safely?

Beginners can safely delve into rope wall practices under expert supervision, gradually acclimating to the techniques and safety protocols.

Are there specific measurements to consider for a personalized rope wall setup?

Customized heights and spatial adjustments are recommended to accommodate individual practitioner needs and enhance comfort during practice.

How do yoga wall ropes differ from traditional yoga practice?

Yoga wall ropes utilize gravity for resistance, facilitating deeper postures and promoting joint relief, distinguishing them from traditional yoga practices.

Yoga Wall Ropes present a transformative approach to yoga, unlocking profound health benefits by integrating gravity and sophisticated setups. Embrace this technique under expert guidance to embark on a holistic journey fostering joint health, mental tranquility, and muscular well-being.

Elevate Your Yoga Practice with Rope Wall Yoga
Unleashing the Power of Rope Wall Yoga

Rope wall yoga, also known as Yoga Kurunta, is a distinctive approach to practicing Iyengar style asanas by utilizing ropes affixed to a wall. This practice, akin to a puppet or doll made of wood, empowers practitioners to explore a new dimension of yoga by suspending themselves from ropes, redefining the boundaries of traditional postures.

The Legacy and Origin

A Gift from B.K.S. Iyengar

The genesis of the rope wall traces back to the ingenuity of B.K.S. Iyengar, evolving from the modest setting of an average Indian dwelling. The utilization of simple ropes, initially secured from standard window gates, paved the way for practitioners to delve deeper into various poses, finding stability and support through rope suspension.

Facilitating All Levels of Practice

Echoing Geeta S. Iyengar's insights, the rope wall emerges as an invaluable tool, particularly aiding individuals grappling with stiffness, weakness, or challenges in executing specific asanas. It acts as a supportive ally, enabling individuals to embrace postures that might otherwise be inaccessible.

Five Compelling Reasons to Embrace Rope Wall Yoga

1. A Novel Perspective on Asanas

Discover an innovative dimension in yoga practice, redefining familiar poses like backbends, forward bends, twists, and inversions. The ropes serve as physical conduits, directing the body and mind towards equilibrium and harmony.

2. Access Deeper Stretches and Strengthening

Leverage the ropes' traction to access areas of the spine that traditional practices might overlook. Dive into challenging asanas like Shoulder Stand and Plow with increased safety and explore enhanced variations of poses like Cobra, facilitating profound chest opening and shoulder release.

3. Prolonged and Supported Asana Experience

With the body secured by ropes and feet anchored, postures such as Downward Facing Dog and Headstand can be sustained for extended periods. This prolonged practice fosters refined breathing techniques and offers substantial benefits for lower back health and inversion experiences.

4. Enhance Mobility and Fluidity

Experience heightened joint mobility beyond regular ranges of motion. The rhythmic momentum of movements, such as transitioning from Cobra Pose to Upward Facing Forward Fold, cultivates agility, concentration, and lightness.

5. Embrace Long-Term Benefits

The allure of rope wall yoga extends beyond immediate results. Regular practice instills patience, discipline, and a sense of suppleness, leaving practitioners walking taller and feeling more resilient in their spine.

Frequently Asked Questions

How Often Should One Practice Rope Wall Yoga?

Consistency and regularity are key. Aim for at least one to two sessions per week to experience progressive benefits and growth in your practice.

Is Rope Wall Yoga Suitable for Beginners?

Absolutely. With proper guidance from seasoned instructors, beginners can safely embark on rope wall yoga, gradually acclimating to the techniques and postures.

Are There Any Precautions to Consider?

Always practice under the guidance of an experienced teacher to ensure safety and prevent undue strain or injury while exploring new postures.

Can Rope Wall Yoga be Practiced at Home?

While many studios offer rope wall setups, practicing at home necessitates proper installation and safety measures. Seek professional guidance if setting up a rope wall at home.

Conclusion

Rope wall yoga represents an evolution in the traditional yoga landscape, offering practitioners a gateway to heightened flexibility, strength, and balance. Embrace this practice under the tutelage of knowledgeable instructors to unlock its full potential and enjoy its myriad benefits.

Exploring the 12 Best Wall Rope Yoga Poses and Their Multifaceted Benefits

Wall Rope Yoga: A Holistic Approach

Wall Rope Yoga is a dynamic practice intertwining traditional yoga with innovative elements. Harnessing the power of wall ropes, this practice offers a unique spectrum of yoga poses, each delivering profound benefits to the body, mind, and spirit.

1. The Revitalizing Inversion: Shoulder Stand

Benefits:

Encourages blood circulation to the brain

Stimulates thyroid gland, aiding metabolism

Relieves stress and calms the nervous system

How to Practice:

Detailed guide on safely executing the Shoulder Stand using wall ropes

2. Balancing Act: Headstand (Sirsasana)

Benefits:

Enhances focus and concentration

Strengthens core muscles and improves balance

Boosts energy levels and alleviates mental fatigue

How to Practice:

Step-by-step instructions for achieving the Headstand with wall rope support

3. Spinal Elevation: Cobra Pose (Bhujangasana)

Benefits:

Expands chest, aiding in deep breathing

Alleviates lower back pain

Strengthens spine and improves posture

How to Practice:

Comprehensive guidance on practicing Cobra Pose using wall ropes

4. The Soothing Plow: Plow Pose (Halasana)

Benefits:

Stretches and relaxes the spine

Calms the nervous system, promoting relaxation

Stimulates abdominal organs, aiding digestion

How to Practice:

Step-by-step instructions for safely adopting the Plow Pose with wall rope assistance

5. Relaxing Forward Fold: Forward Fold (Urdhva Mukha Paschimottanasana)

Benefits:

Stretches hamstrings and back muscles

Reduces stress and anxiety

Enhances flexibility and eases tension in the body

How to Practice:

Detailed guide to performing Forward Fold using wall ropes for support

6. The Strengthening Bridge: Bridge Pose (Setu Bandhasana)

Benefits:

Strengthens back, glutes, and hamstrings

Opens up the chest, aiding in better breathing

Relieves lower back pain and fatigue

How to Practice:

Step-by-step instructions for achieving the Bridge Pose with wall rope assistance

7. The Stability Enhancer: Tree Pose (Vrksasana)

Benefits:

Enhances balance and stability

Strengthens legs, ankles, and feet

Improves concentration and mental focus

How to Practice:

Detailed guidance on practicing Tree Pose utilizing wall ropes

8. The Grounding Warrior: Warrior Pose (Virabhadrasana)

Benefits:

Strengthens legs, arms, and core

Enhances focus and determination

Improves circulation and respiration

How to Practice:

Comprehensive instructions for achieving the Warrior Pose with wall rope support

9. The Twisting Detox: Revolved Triangle Pose (Parivrtta Trikonasana)

Benefits:

Stimulates abdominal organs, aiding digestion

Stretches and tones abdominal muscles

Detoxifies and energizes the body

How to Practice:

Step-by-step guidance on practicing the Revolved Triangle Pose using wall ropes

10. The Balancing Act Redux: Extended Hand-to-Big-Toe Pose (Utthita Hasta Padangusthasana)

Benefits:

Improves balance and focus

Strengthens ankles and legs

Stretches hamstrings and hip flexors

How to Practice:

Detailed guide to achieving the Extended Hand-to-Big-Toe Pose with wall rope assistance

11. The Restorative Child: Child's Pose (Balasana)

Benefits:

Relieves tension in the back, shoulders, and chest

Promotes relaxation and stress relief

Stretches and lengthens the spine

How to Practice:

Step-by-step instructions for safely adopting the Child's Pose using wall ropes

12. The Stretching Triangle: Triangle Pose (Trikonasana)

Benefits:

Strengthens legs, arms, and core

Stretches hamstrings and hips

Opens up chest and shoulders

How to Practice:

Comprehensive guidance on practicing the Triangle Pose utilizing wall ropes

Frequently Asked Questions

Q: Can beginners practice Wall Rope Yoga Poses?

A: Yes, beginners can start under the guidance of a certified instructor and gradually progress to more complex poses.

Q: How often should one practice these poses?

A: Consistent practice, even a few times a week, can yield benefits. However, it's crucial to listen to your body and avoid overexertion.

Q: Are these poses suitable for individuals with prior injuries?

A: It's advisable to consult a healthcare professional before starting any new exercise routine, especially if one has existing injuries or health concerns.

Immerse yourself in the transformative world of Wall Rope Yoga, embracing these 12 invigorating poses and unlocking a journey of holistic wellness and vitality.

Wall Rope Yoga May Sound Intimidating, But It's Amazing for the Body—Here's Everything You Benefits

Wall Rope Yoga: A Holistic Approach

Wall Rope Yoga is a dynamic practice intertwining traditional yoga with innovative elements. Harnessing the power of wall ropes, this practice offers a unique spectrum of yoga poses, each delivering profound benefits to the body, mind, and spirit.

1. The Revitalizing Inversion: Shoulder Stand

Benefits:

Encourages blood circulation to the brain

Stimulates thyroid gland, aiding metabolism

Relieves stress and calms the nervous system

How to Practice:

Detailed guide on safely executing the Shoulder Stand using wall ropes

2. Balancing Act: Headstand (Sirsasana)

Benefits:

Enhances focus and concentration

Strengthens core muscles and improves balance

Boosts energy levels and alleviates mental fatigue

How to Practice:

Step-by-step instructions for achieving the Headstand with wall rope support

3. Spinal Elevation: Cobra Pose (Bhujangasana)

Benefits:

Expands chest, aiding in deep breathing

Alleviates lower back pain

Strengthens spine and improves posture

How to Practice:

Comprehensive guidance on practicing Cobra Pose using wall ropes

4. The Soothing Plow: Plow Pose (Halasana)

Benefits:

Stretches and relaxes the spine

Calms the nervous system, promoting relaxation

Stimulates abdominal organs, aiding digestion

How to Practice:

Step-by-step instructions for safely adopting the Plow Pose with wall rope assistance

5. Relaxing Forward Fold: Forward Fold (Urdhva Mukha Paschimottanasana)

Benefits:

Stretches hamstrings and back muscles

Reduces stress and anxiety

Enhances flexibility and eases tension in the body

How to Practice:

Detailed guide to performing Forward Fold using wall ropes for support

6. The Strengthening Bridge: Bridge Pose (Setu Bandhasana)

Benefits:

Strengthens back, glutes, and hamstrings

Opens up the chest, aiding in better breathing

Relieves lower back pain and fatigue

How to Practice:

Step-by-step instructions for achieving the Bridge Pose with wall rope assistance

7. The Stability Enhancer: Tree Pose (Vrksasana)

Benefits:

Enhances balance and stability

Strengthens legs, ankles, and feet

Improves concentration and mental focus

How to Practice:

Detailed guidance on practicing Tree Pose utilizing wall ropes

8. The Grounding Warrior: Warrior Pose (Virabhadrasana)

Benefits:

Strengthens legs, arms, and core

Enhances focus and determination

Improves circulation and respiration

How to Practice:

Comprehensive instructions for achieving the Warrior Pose with wall rope support

9. The Twisting Detox: Revolved Triangle Pose (Parivrtta Trikonasana)

Benefits:

Stimulates abdominal organs, aiding digestion

Stretches and tones abdominal muscles

Detoxifies and energizes the body

How to Practice:

Step-by-step guidance on practicing the Revolved Triangle Pose using wall ropes

10. The Balancing Act Redux: Extended Hand-to-Big-Toe Pose (Utthita Hasta Padangusthasana)

Benefits:

Improves balance and focus

Strengthens ankles and legs

Stretches hamstrings and hip flexors

How to Practice:

Detailed guide to achieving the Extended Hand-to-Big-Toe Pose with wall rope assistance

11. The Restorative Child: Child's Pose (Balasana)

Benefits:

Relieves tension in the back, shoulders, and chest

Promotes relaxation and stress relief

Stretches and lengthens the spine

How to Practice:

Step-by-step instructions for safely adopting the Child's Pose using wall ropes

12. The Stretching Triangle: Triangle Pose (Trikonasana)

Benefits:

Strengthens legs, arms, and core

Stretches hamstrings and hips

Opens up chest and shoulders

How to Practice:

Comprehensive guidance on practicing the Triangle Pose utilizing wall ropes

Frequently Asked Questions

Q: Can beginners practice Wall Rope Yoga Poses?

A: Yes, beginners can start under the guidance of a certified instructor and gradually progress to more complex poses.

Q: How often should one practice these poses?

A: Consistent practice, even a few times a week, can yield benefits. However, it's crucial to listen to your body and avoid overexertion.

Q: Are these poses suitable for individuals with prior injuries?

A: It's advisable to consult a healthcare professional before starting any new exercise routine, especially if one has existing injuries or health concerns.

Immerse yourself in the transformative world of Wall Rope Yoga, embracing these 12 invigorating poses and unlocking a journey of holistic wellness and vitality.

Wall Rope Yoga May Sound Intimidating, But It's Amazing for the Body—Here's Everything You Need to Know

Wall Rope Yoga: A Comprehensive Guide for Exploring Its Benefits

Understanding Wall Rope Yoga

Wall Rope Yoga might seem daunting initially, but its benefits for the body and mind are unparalleled. This holistic practice integrates traditional yoga with the assistance of wall ropes, offering a unique approach to enhancing overall well-being.

Unveiling the Essence of Wall Rope Yoga

Wall Rope Yoga Origins

Wall Rope Yoga, often associated with Iyengar Yoga, utilizes ropes anchored to a wall to aid practitioners in executing various yoga poses with precision and support. This approach allows individuals to delve deeper into poses and experience profound benefits.

Benefits of Wall Rope Yoga

Enhanced Precision: The ropes serve as guides, aiding in achieving correct alignment and posture.

Deeper Stretches: Assistance from the ropes allows for deeper stretches, benefiting muscles and joints.

Balanced Support: Practitioners, irrespective of experience, find support in complex poses, enhancing confidence and stability.

Targeted Muscle Engagement: Specific muscles are activated and strengthened with the added resistance provided by the ropes.

Mind-Body Harmony: The practice cultivates a deeper mind-body connection through controlled movements and breathing.

Exploring Key Wall Rope Yoga Poses

1. Shoulder Stand with Wall Ropes

Benefits:

Improved blood circulation

Stimulated thyroid gland

Stress relief and nervous system calming

2. Headstand (Sirsasana)

Benefits:

Enhanced focus and balance

Boosted energy levels

Improved core strength

3. Cobra Pose (Bhujangasana)

Benefits:

Expanded chest for deeper breathing

Alleviated lower back pain

Improved posture

Frequently Asked Questions

Q: Is Wall Rope Yoga suitable for beginners?

A: Yes, beginners can start with proper guidance from a certified instructor to understand the techniques and progress gradually.

Q: Can Wall Rope Yoga help with flexibility?

A: Absolutely. The practice enables deeper stretches, enhancing overall flexibility over time.

Q: How often should one practice Wall Rope Yoga?

A: Consistency is key. Practicing a few times a week can yield significant benefits, but it's crucial to respect one's body and avoid overexertion.

Embark on Your Wall Rope Yoga Journey

Wall Rope Yoga, though initially intimidating, offers a gateway to enriching the body and mind. Dive into this practice with guidance, explore the poses, and witness the transformation.

Affordable and adaptable Iyengar yoga series for home practice

This series of simple Iyengar yoga poses are perfect to start your Iyengar yoga practice. It focuses primarily on standing poses and includes several inversions that are essential to the Iyengar yoga sequence. The inverted pose is designed for advanced students and can easily be skipped for beginners. You don't have to worry about extra yoga gear. A yoga mat and some blocks are nice to bring, but not necessary. This personalized series allows you to easily enter the world of Iyengar Yoga online or at home.

Iyengar yoga sequence

If you want to find more information and resources about the Iyengar yoga sequence, including variations and modifications, Yoga Selection is a great online platform to explore. Yoga Choice offers extensive guidance and instructional videos to support your Iyengar yoga

practice at home or wherever you
are.

Uttanasana Iyengar yoga pose

Stand with your feet hip-width
apart and the insides of your feet
parallel. Lower your arms and
place your hands on the floor or on
your shins. Relax your neck and
lower your head, but lift and
broaden your shoulders. Keep
your knees straight and your hips
directly over your ankles.

Extend the front of your body
while straightening the back of
your body. Go deeper

Partially bend your knees (about
15° from vertical).

Bend your knees and rotate so that your kneecap points forward. Bend your knees forward...and press into the base of your big toe and heel bone at the same time.

Continue these movements by straightening your legs again. Make sure your knees are straight forward.

Iyengar yoga downward facing dog pose

Adho Mukha Svanasana

Place your hands shoulder-width apart on the floor. Bend and extend your toes so that they point forward.

Place your feet hip-width apart. Twist so that your toes are pointing forward.

Keep enough distance between your legs and arms so that your body forms a right angle when viewed from the side. Go deeper

As in the previous position, partially bend your knees.

Partially bend your knees and consciously adjust the angle of your knees so that they point straight ahead. Slowly straighten your legs again without breaking the angle of your knees. As you straighten your legs again, notice the general tendency of your legs to roll in or out. Once the legs are straight, press the area above and below the knee back with equal force.

Now press your upper pelvis and the back of your lower leg with the same force.

Trikonasana Iyengar Yoga

Trikonasana

Place your left heel against the wall and your right foot away from the wall. Make sure your feet are about a foot apart. Turn your left foot in and your right foot out.

Align your right heel with your left arch. Reach your right hand toward the ground or shin.

Raise your arms up. Go deeper

Bend your right knee in half and look at your right leg.

Bend your right knee in half and press the base of your right big toe firmly into the floor. Applying pressure on the base of the thumbs, rotate the patella so that they point to the sides.

Keep your hip straight toward the front of your body. While doing the above movement, slowly straighten your legs again, being careful not to extend your knees to the sides.

Bend your knees to the sides, point your chest and face toward the ceiling, and look up with your thumbs up.

Virabhadrasana 2 Iyengar yoga

With your left heel touching the wall, step your right foot about a foot away.

When bending the front leg, make sure the knee is in line with the ankle. Extend your right arm out to the side so that the shoulder is at the level of the wrist and the palm is facing down.

With your front leg bent, touch the wall with your left toes. Go deeper

Instead of bending your right leg in one continuous motion, bend your right leg in half.

Bend your leg in half, increase the pressure on your right heel, and rotate your inner knee at your hip. As you do this, keep your hip straight facing the front of your body.

As above, continue to bend your right leg until your upper thigh is parallel to the floor. In this position, stretch your legs straight from your hips to the inside of your knees.

At the same time, draw inward from the right outer knee to the outer hip toward the center line of the body.

Parsvakonasana using ribs

Parsvakonasana

Place the ball and heel of your foot on the floor and place your right foot against the wall. The sole angle is 45°. Move the left leg back so that the distance between the legs is slightly greater than the length of the legs.

Place your right hand on the floor or next to your right outer leg. Make sure your right hand is touching the outside of your right knee.

Place your left toes on the wall just above your right foot. The elbows are bent straight towards the upper ceiling.

Go deeper

Press the base of your right finger firmly into the wall. Press your right knee firmly into your right hand. Resist this pressure with your hands. Rotate your chest toward the ceiling.

Pull your right hip back into your hip socket. Move your arms back along the wall to improve chest rotation.

To further improve chest rotation, press your left heel harder into the floor.

Ardha Chandrasana Iyengar Yoga

Stand on your right leg and press your left leg against the wall.

Place your right hand on the floor just below your right shoulder. If you can't reach the ground without bending your knees, use a block in your hand.

Make sure your right wrist is under your right hip. Extend your upper arms up and place your wrists on your shoulders.

Go deeper

Partially bend your right knee. Bend your right knee and rotate it straight to the side.

At the same time, lift your right hip toward your buttocks and turn back toward the wall. Twist your kneecap to the side and maintain the lift in your right hip as you slowly straighten your leg again.

Press your left heel harder into the wall. Lift your left inner knee.

Keep your left hip toward your thigh. Roll your chest toward the ceiling and look at your toes.

Parivrta Ardha Chandrasana
Engar Yoga

Place your left foot against the wall so that your ankle is in line with your thigh. Stand on your right leg with your ankle under your right thigh.

Place both hands on the floor just below your shoulders. Use blocks under the arms if necessary.

Look at your upper leg and make sure your toes are pointing straight down. Place your left hand on the floor (or block) and bring your right hand to your right hip.

Roll your left shoulder down and your right shoulder up. Raise your right hand to the ceiling.

Turn your head and look at the tip of your thumb. Go deeper

Press your left heel harder into the wall.

Lift your left hip. Twist your left hip over your right hip without lowering your left hip.

Without lowering your left hip, straighten your left back and twist your body toward the floor. Bend your left back toward the floor.

Lift and point the inside of your left foot against the wall. Extend the left side of your spine away from your ribs.

Parivrta Trikonasana Iyengar Yoga

Place your left heel against the wall and turn your foot deep inward. Extend your right leg one leg longer than your left leg.

Bring your left hand to the outside of your right leg. Use a block in your hand if necessary.

Bring your right hand to your right hip. Roll your left shoulder down and your right shoulder up at the same time.

He turns his head and looks up. Stretch your arms up.

Go deeper

In the position described above, turn your head so that you can see your right leg. Keep looking down and center your face on the inside of your right leg.

Press the inside of your right foot firmly into the floor. Keeping pressure on your inner foot on the floor, rotate your right hip toward the wall behind you.

Straighten your back to the left and twist towards the floor. Bend your left back toward the floor.

Press your left hand harder into the ground (or block) and move your left shoulder blade deeper into your body. Once the rotation of the lower back, ribs and shoulders is evident, turn your gaze to the tip of the thumb.

Parivrta Parsvakonasana

Place your left heel against the wall. Lift your right leg away from the wall.

Bend your right leg and make sure your knee is aligned vertically over your ankle. If necessary, adjust the distance between the legs to align them.

Bring your left shoulder over your right knee, covering the space between your armpit and knee. Roll your left shoulder down and your right shoulder up at the same time.

Raise your arm and then towards you. Go deeper

Press your inner right heel harder into the ground, relaxing your right inner thigh as you do so.

Release the right hip down. Vigorously lift your left shin without lifting your hips.

Place your left heel against the wall and rotate the inside of your left foot away from the floor. Relax your right inner thigh and move your pelvis toward your right hip.

Rotate your left hip outward from your right hip. Straighten your back to the left and twist down.

The left wall has collapsed. Lean the outer side of your right thigh against the wall and move your sternum toward your neck.

Place your back leg against the wall and stretch it out. Move your lumbar spine toward your skull.

Move your back leg and upper arm in opposite directions.

Virabhadrasana using ribs

Step on the ball of your right foot at a 45° angle to the wall.

Move your left foot back and away from the wall. The distance between the legs should be slightly more than the length of one leg.

Place your fingers on a wall at chest height. Keep your left leg straight and bend your right leg.

Go deeper

When you bend your right leg, make sure the knee is pointing straight ahead.

Extend your right inner knee outward while simultaneously pulling your outer knee to the outside of your thigh. Rotate your left hip outward from your right hip.

Twist the front of your pelvis to the right. Then lift and straighten the inside of your left leg.

Without lowering your back knee, lower your glutes and lift your hips. Press your fingertips firmly into the wall and lift your sternum away from your stomach.

Virabhadrasana 3

Start in a half-dog position with your toes touching the wall at hip height. Stand with your feet together and your ankles under your thighs.

Lift the left leg, straighten the knee and bring the bottom to the level of the ankle. Go deeper

Lift your left leg without lowering your right hip.

Bend your left hip down. Lift your left inner thigh.

Rotate your left hip outward from your right hip. Raise both elbows while keeping your chest on the floor.

Lift your belly without lowering your back legs. Press your toes firmly into the wall and extend the inside of your left leg away from the wall.

Parsvottanasana

Place your left heel against the wall and turn your foot deep inward. Lift your right leg away from the wall and move your feet so that they are about 1 foot apart.

Start with your hands on your hips. Keep your chest open as you place your hands on the ground on either side of your right leg. Put your hand on the block if necessary. Go deeper

Press the inner edge of your right foot firmly into the floor.

Pull the thigh of your right leg up and back. Rotate your left hip outward from your right hip.

Turn the boat from left to right. Straighten your back to the left and twist down.

Stabilize your right hip and shift your pelvis toward your right hip. Place your hand on your left leg and repeat. When using blocks, hold them in your hand. Bring your chest, not your face, to your right leg.

Prasarita Padottanasana Iyengar Yoga

Place the outer edge of one leg against the wall. The ribs support your legs and help keep them straight.

Place your other leg slightly longer than the length of your leg. Make sure the insides of your feet are parallel.

Place your hands on the floor just below your shoulders with your spine open. Use a block in your hand if necessary.

Move your arms back, bend your elbows and keep your hands on the floor. Point your fingers in the same direction as your toes.

He lowers his head to the floor. Go deeper

Press into the outer edges of your legs and lift your shins into the lips of your hips.

Turn the inside of the finger down. Pull your outer elbow back.

Raise your shoulders. Extend your trapezius muscles outward.

Lower the skin of the waist. Gently ease your belly toward your spine.

Sirsasana (headrest)

When you balance, place more of your weight in the center of each ankle. Press your wrists down and lift your shoulder sockets.

At the same time, straighten and lift the shoulder blades. Move the muscles from the sides of the ribcage to the front of the body.

Lift the sides of the ribcage without letting the front of the ribs bend outward.

Lift the sides of your hips without letting the back of your hips drop. Bend your groin back and move your tailbone toward the groin.

Lift and stretch from the inside of the groin to the inside of the heel. Setu Bandha Sarvangasana

Place a high block on your sacrum. Rotate the block so the width of the block goes across the back of your thigh to widen your thighs. Adjust the distance from the block to the wall so you can bring your feet up the wall so your ankles are at hip level.

Make sure the inner heel is firmly against the wall. Make sure your shoulders touch the floor.

Hold the front of your hips so the block helps lift the back of your hips. Leave your stomach empty.

Lift the part of the spine between the shoulder blades. Lift your armpits.

Relax your throat, tongue and eyes. Watch your breathing become softer and smoother.

Savasana

Let the back of your pelvis pull toward the floor. Pull your front hips toward your back hips.

Encourage your abdomen to relax down with each exhalation. Make sure your chest has room to rise and expand as you inhale, without taking deep breaths.

Your eyes and temples will feel relaxed.